# VEGAN DIET COOKBOOK FOR SENIOR

## The complete 25 easy and healthy recipes to strengthen your immune system

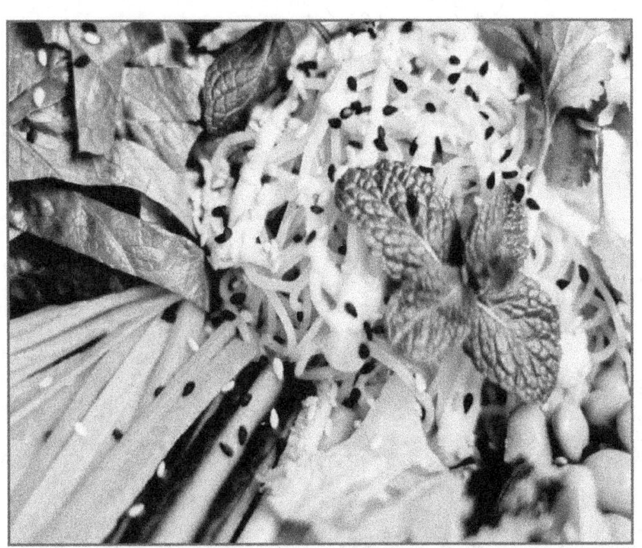

## Reina W. Edwonds

# COPYRIGHT
## All right reserved

No part of this publication may be reproduced by, distributed, or transmitted in any form or by any means, including photocopying, recording, or other electronic or mechanical methods, without the prior written permission of the publisher, except in the case of brief quotations embodies in critical reviews and certain other noncommercial uses permitted by copyright law

**Copyright @ 2024  by Reina W. Edwonds**

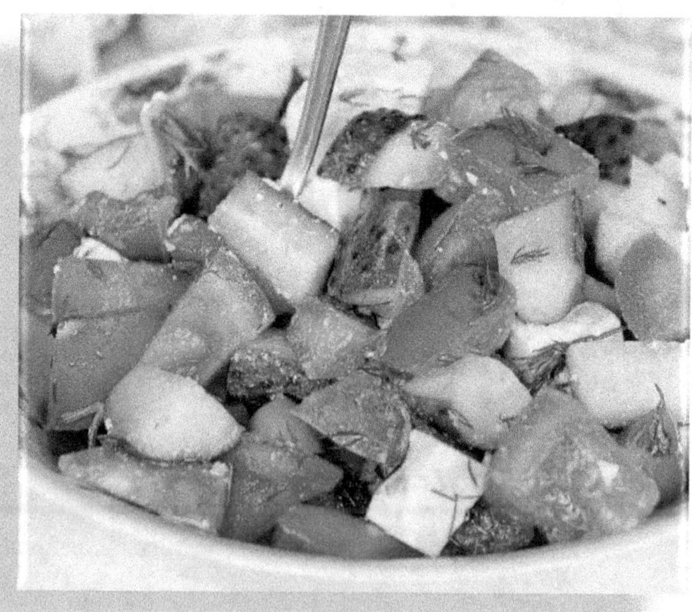

# TABLE OF CONTENT

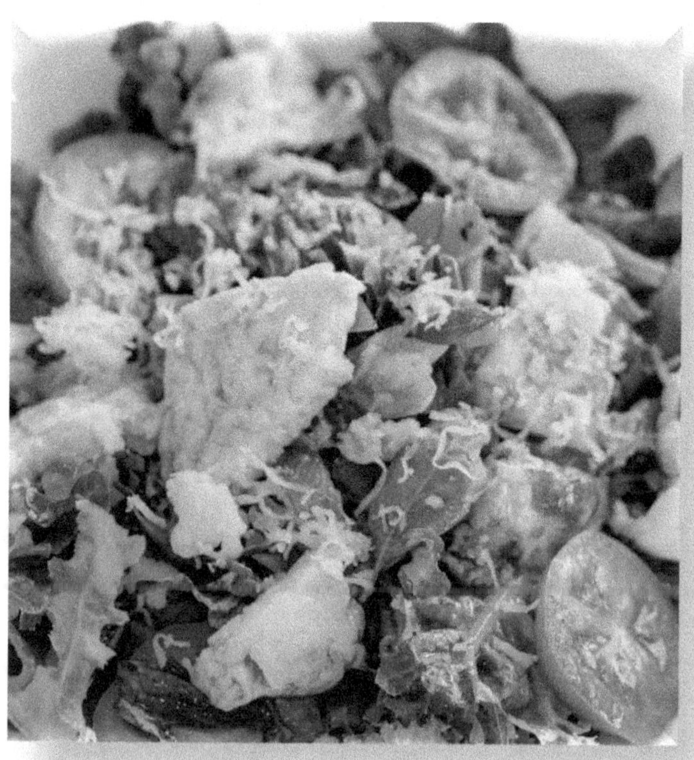

# INTRODUCTION

Clara, an elderly woman with a heart as strong as the hills surrounding her, resided in the peaceful village of Greenhaven, where the breeze carried the aroma of growing flowers. Her days were spent with Henry, a companion through the seasons, and their small house was filled with anecdotes of a life well lived.

As the light warmed Greenhaven, Clara and Henry felt the subtle tug of time. The light that had once powered their days dimmed, and Clara wished there was a way to regain the vitality that had slid away so elegantly.

Clara discovered a world of possibilities one day while reading an old book: a vegan diet promising vigour and a fresh attitude. As she shared this revelation with Henry, she was filled with excitement, expecting it would give their golden years fresh meaning.

However, the perfume of traditional dinners stayed in Clara's mind, a comfortable reminder of the past. Clara hesitated, unsure whether taking this new route meant saying goodbye to the rich flavours that had seasoned their shared meals. Henry calmed her with a soft smile and encouraging words, and they agreed to go on this gastronomic journey together.

Clara and Henry sowed the seeds of transformation in the heart of Greenhaven, where flowers adorn the landscape. The delicacies that had previously graced their table had morphed into a brilliant tapestry of plant-based pleasures, sustaining not just their bodies but also the undying love that had survived the years. Change blossomed in the garden of their life, ushering in a new chapter in their shared tale.

# CHAPTER 1: Nutritional Guildlines For Senior Vegans

In the fabric of time, where the chapters of life develop, the dietary requirements for elderly vegans sound like a symphony of energy. Each note, a carefully constructed tune, conveys the spirit of well-being amid the golden years.

## Essential Nutrients for Nourishing Wisdom

Wisdom emerges when basic nutrients are in balance. It's a ballet of vitamins and minerals, a lyrical interaction that powers the body's orchestra. As seniors embrace this nutritional dance, they discover power in the rhythm of plant-based nourishment.

## Plant Nutrient Sources: Nature's Abundance

In the embrace of nature's riches, the senior vegan experiences a spiritual feast. Every meal, from the vivid colours of veggies to the sustaining power of legumes, is a stroke on the health canvas. The garden of plant-based nutrients becomes a haven, providing nourishment and strength.

## Meal Planning Tips for Seniors: Crafting Wellness

Meal preparation for seniors goes beyond the kitchen; it's an art form that cultivates wellbeing. It's about enjoying the simplicity of a carefully chosen meal that considers balance and flavour. This gastronomic adventure provides seniors with more than just nutrition; it is also a celebration of life's flavours.

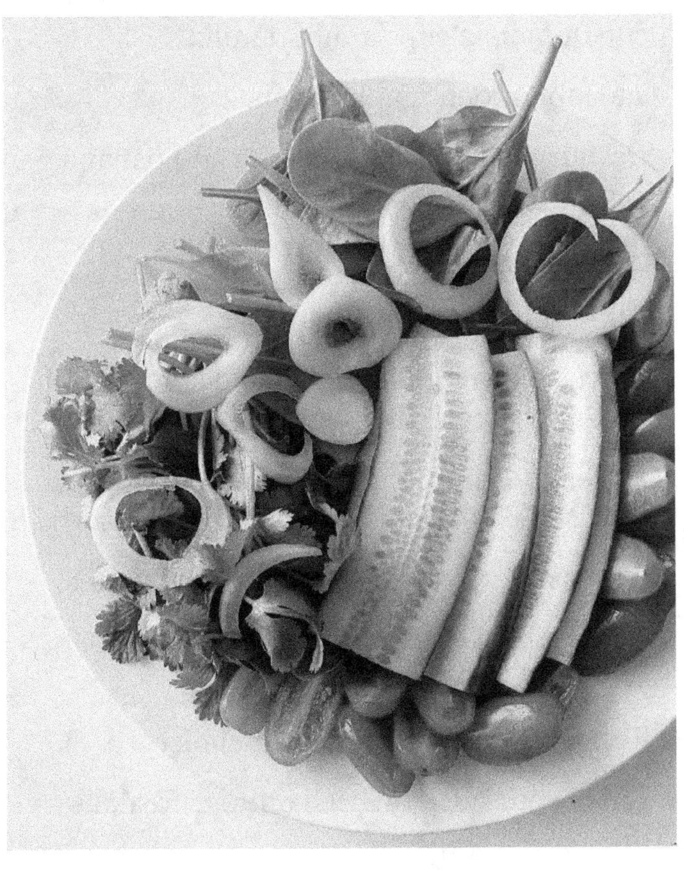

# CHAPTER 2: Breakfast Recipes

## *1. Breakfast Bowl Made With Quinoa*

### Ingredients:

1 cup quinoa, 2 cups almond milk.

- One tablespoon maple syrup.

- Fresh fruits (e.g., strawberries and banana slices).

### Preparation:

1. Rinse the quinoa in cool water.

2. In a saucepan, mix quinoa and almond milk. Heat until it boils, then lower to a simmer.

3. Cover and simmer for 15 minutes, or until the quinoa is soft and liquid has been absorbed.

4. Add maple syrup and cover for 5 minutes.

5. Fluff quinoa with a fork and divide among bowls.

6. Top with fresh fruits of your choice.

7. Enjoy your nutrient-rich quinoa breakfast dish!

**Cooking time:** 20 minutes

## 2. Chia Seed Pudding with Berries

**Ingredients:**

- 1/4 cup Chia seeds

 1 cup almond milk,

1 tablespoon agave syrup.

- mixed berries (strawberries and blueberries)

**Preparation:**

1. In a mixing dish, combine chia seeds, almond milk, and agave syrup.

2. Stir thoroughly, cover, and refrigerate for at least 4 hours or overnight.

3. Stir again before serving for a pudding-like consistency.

4. Transfer to serving platters or jars.

5. Sprinkle with mixed berries.

6. Serve cool.

7. Indulge in your scrumptious chia seed pudding!

**Cooking Time:** overnight or four hours

## *3. Vegan muesli with almond milk.*

### Ingredients:

1 cup rolled oats,

2 cups almond milk,

1 tablespoon nut butter.

- Top with sliced bananas or almonds.

### Preparation:

1. In a saucepan, combine the almond milk and rolled oats.

2. Bring to a mild boil, then turn the heat down to low.

3. Simmer for 5-7 minutes, stirring regularly, until the oats become creamy.

4. Mix in the nut butter.

5. Take it off the heat and let it rest for one minute.

6. Transfer to dishes and top with sliced bananas or almonds.

7. Your warm and soothing vegan muesli is ready to be consumed!

**<u>Cooking Time</u>**: 10 Minutes

## *4. Avocado Toast with Tomato*

### **<u>Ingredients:</u>**

- Two pieces of whole grain bread - One ripe avocado

Cherry tomatoes, sliced

- Add Season with salt and pepper as desired.

### **<u>Preparation:</u>**

1. Toast the whole-grain bread pieces.

2. In a bowl, mash the ripe avocado while it toasts.

3. Spread the mashed avocado equally on the toasted bread.

4. Garnish with sliced cherry tomatoes.

5. Add salt and pepper to taste.

6. Serve immediately as a quick and nutritious breakfast.

7. Embrace the simplicity of avocado toast!

**<u>Cooking time</u>**: 5 minutes

## *5. Banana Pancakes are vegan.*

### **Ingredients:**

 1 cup flour,

1 tablespoon sugar,

1 tablespoon baking powder.

- One cup of almond milk

- 1 ripe, mashed banana

### **Preparation:**

1. Combine flour, sugar, and baking powder in a mixing basin.

2. Add the almond milk and mashed bananas. Stir until just mixed.

3. Heat a nonstick skillet on medium heat.

4. Pour 1/4 cup batter for each pancake into the skillet.

5. Cook until bubbles appear on the surface, then turn and cook on the other side.

6. Repeat until all of the batter has been utilised.

7. Top your fluffy vegan banana pancakes with your preferred toppings.

**Cooking time**: 15 minutes

# CHAPTER 3: Lunch Recipes

## *1. Lentil and Vegetable Soup.*

**Ingredients:**

-1 cup lentils

- 4 cups vegetable broth - 1 sliced onion

2 sliced carrots and 2 cut celery stalks.

- 2 cloves of minced garlic

1 teaspoon cumin, salt, and pepper to taste.

**<u>Preparation:</u>**

1. Rinse the lentils with cool water.

2. In a large saucepan, cook the onions, carrots, and celery until softened.

3. Cook for another minute with the garlic and cumin.

4. Pour in vegetable broth and lentils.

5. Bring to a boil, then decrease heat and let simmer for 20-25 minutes.

6. Sprinkle with salt and pepper.

7. Serve hot and savour your delicious lentil and vegetable soup!

## *2. Chickpea Salad Wraps.*

### Ingredients:

- 1 can drained and rinsed chickpea

s - 1/2 cup diced cucumber

- 1/2 cup cherry tomatoes, halved

- 1/4 cup finely chopped red onion - Fresh parsley, chopped

- 2 tablespoons olive oil

- Lemon juice to taste - Salt and pepper to taste - Whole grain wraps

### Preparation:

1. In a mixing dish, add chickpeas, cucumbers, tomatoes, red onion, and parsley.

2. Drizzle the mixture with olive oil and lemon juice.

3. Season with salt and pepper, then toss to mix.

4. Serve the chickpea salad on whole-grain wraps.

5. Roll into wraps and fasten with toothpicks.

6. Slice in half and serve.

7. Enjoy your cool chickpea salad wraps!

**<u>Cooking Time:</u>** 15 Minutes


## *3. Sweet Potato and Kale Salad.*

**<u>Ingredients:</u>**

- 2 diced sweet potatoes

- 1 bunch chopped kale (stems removed) –

1/4 cup dried cranberries

- 1/4 cup pumpkin seeds.

- Two teaspoons of balsamic vinaigrette

- Season with salt and pepper to taste.

**<u>Preparation:</u>**

1. Place sweet potato cubes in the oven until cooked.

2. Massage kale with a pinch of salt until tender.

3. In a large mixing basin, add the kale, sweet potatoes, dried cranberries, and pumpkin seeds.

4. Toss salad with balsamic vinaigrette.

5. Season with salt and pepper as desired.

6. Serve at ambient temperature.

7. Enjoy the delicious sweet potato and kale salad!

**Cooking time**: 25 minutes


## *4. Vegan Buddha Bowl*

**Ingredients:**

cooked quinoa and canned,

 drained chickpeas.

- Sliced avocado - Shredded carrots.

Cucumber, sliced

- Hummus with lemon tahini dressing.

**Preparation:**

1. Form the bowl's foundation with cooked quinoa.

2. Divide chickpeas, avocado, shredded carrots, and cucumber into sections.

3. Spread hummus in one part.

4. Drizzle with lemon tahini dressing.

5. Serve immediately, combining the ingredients as desired.

6. Enjoy the bright colours and flavours.

7. Your vegan Buddha bowl is ready to be consumed!

**Cooking Time:** 15 Minutes

## *5. Quinoa Stuffed Bell Peppers.*

**Ingredients:**

- Four bell peppers should be sliced in half then removed the  seeds. - Cook one cup of quinoa.

- 1 can black beans, drained and rinsed - 1 cup corn kernels.

- 1 cup salsa.

- Add 1 teaspoon cumin and 1 teaspoon chilli powder.

- Vegan cheese (optional).

**Preparation:**

1. Preheat the oven to 375° F (190° C).

2. In a mixing bowl, combine quinoa, black beans, corn, salsa, cumin and chilli powder.

3. Fill the bell pepper halves with the quinoa mixture.

4. If desired, put vegan cheese over top.

5. Arrange filled peppers in a baking tray.

6. Bake for 25 to 30 minutes, or until the peppers are soft.

7. Serve hot and enjoy your delectable quinoa-stuffed bell peppers!

**<u>Cooking time</u>**: 35 minutes

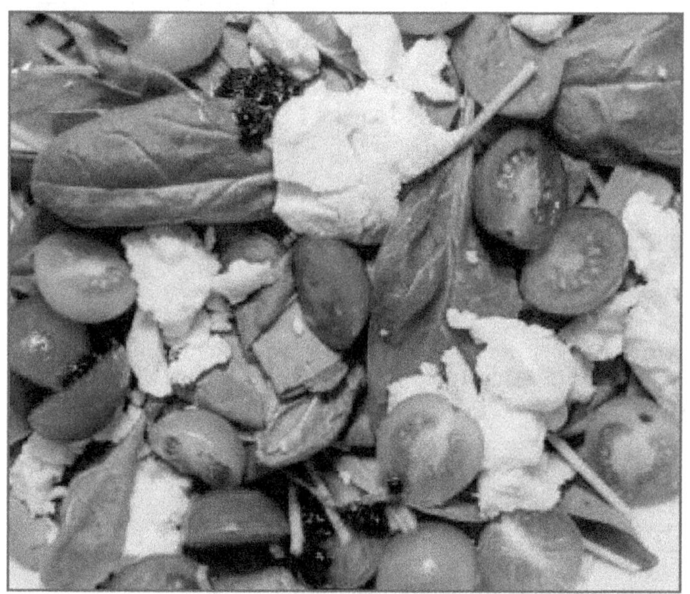

# CHAPTER 4: Dinner Recipes

## *1. Eggplant-Tomato Casserole*

### Ingredients:

- 2 medium-sized eggplants, cut

- 2 cups cherry tomatoes, cut in half

- 1 cup shredded vegan cheese.

- 2 tablespoons of olive oil.

- 2 cloves of minced garlic

- Fresh basil chopped

- Season with salt and pepper to taste.

### Preparation:

1. Preheat the oven to 375° F (190° C).

2. Place eggplant slices in a baking tray.

3. Season the aubergine with minced garlic.

4. Add halved cherry tomatoes on top.

5. Drizzle with olive oil and sprinkle with salt and pepper.

6. Spread the vegan cheese evenly.

7. Bake for 25-30 minutes, until the cheese is melted and bubbling.

8. Top with fresh basil and serve your delicious eggplant and tomato dish!

**Cooking time:** 30 minutes


## *2) Vegan Lentil Loaf*

**Ingredients:**

- One cup of cooked lentils

- One cup of breadcrumbs

Finely chop one onion and mince two garlic cloves.

- One cup of tomato sauce

- 1 tablespoon of soy sauce.

- Add 1 teaspoon dried thyme and season with salt and pepper to taste.

**Preparation:**

1. Preheat the oven to 375° F (190° C).

2. In a mixing bowl, combine cooked lentils, breadcrumbs, diced onion, minced garlic, tomato sauce, soy sauce, dried thyme, salt, and pepper.

3.Pour the mixture into a loaf pan that has been oiled.

4. Bake for 35-40 minutes, until the top is brown.

5. Allow to cool briefly before slicing.

6. Pair your savoury vegan lentil loaf with your favourite sides.

7. Savour your comfortable and nutritious dinner!

**Cooking time:** 40 minutes.


## 3. Spaghetti squash Primavera

**Ingredients:**

- 1 spaghetti squash, halved and seeds removed

- 2 cups mixed veggies (bell peppers, cherry tomatoes, broccoli)

- 2 tablespoons olive oil

- 2 cloves minced garlic

- Fresh parsley chopped

- Season with salt and pepper to taste.

**Preparation:**

1. Preheat the oven to 375° F (190° C).

2. Coat the cut sides of the spaghetti squash with olive oil and season with salt and pepper.

3. Place squash halves on a baking pan, cut side down.

4. Roast for 40–45 minutes, or until the flesh is soft.

5. Sauté minced garlic in olive oil until aromatic.

6. Cook the mixed veggies until tender-crisp.

7. Using a fork, scrape the spaghetti squash into "noodles" and combine with the sautéed veggies.

8. Finish with fresh parsley and serve your delicious spaghetti squash primavera!

**Cooking Time:** 50 Minutes

## 4. Cauliflower and chickpea curry

**Ingredients:**

- One cauliflower sliced into florets.

- Drain and rinse 1 can of chickpeas - Finely slice 1 onion - Add 2 teaspoons curry powder

Ingredients: 1 can coconut milk and 2 teaspoons vegetable oil.

- Chop fresh cilantro - Season with salt and pepper as desired.

## **Preparation:**

1. Heat vegetable oil in a skillet, then sauté chopped onion until softened.

2. Combine cauliflower, chickpeas, and curry powder. Cook for around 5 minutes.

3. Season the coconut milk with salt and pepper.

4. Cook for 20-25 minutes, until the cauliflower is soft.

5. Before serving, garnish with chopped fresh cilantro.

6. Serve your hearty cauliflower and chickpea stew over rice or naan.

**Cooking time:** 30 minutes


## *5. Vegan Shepherd's Pie*

## **Ingredients:**

Ingredients: 4 cups mashed potatoes, 1 cup cooked green lentils, 1 finely chopped onion, 2 diced carrots, 1 cup peas, and 2 tablespoons tomato paste.

- 2 teaspoons of soy sauce.

Ingredients: 2 minced garlic cloves and 2 tablespoons olive oil.

- Season with salt and pepper to taste.

## **Preparation:**

1. Preheat the oven to 375° F (190° C).

2. In a pan, cook the chopped onion and garlic in olive oil until softened.

3. Cook the chopped carrots until soft.

4. Add in the cooked lentils, peas, tomato paste, and soy sauce.

5. Sprinkle with salt and pepper.

6. Add the lentil mixture to a baking dish.

7. Spread the mashed potatoes equally on top.

8. Bake until the top is golden, which should take around 25-30 minutes.

9. Serve your delicious vegan shepherd's pie fresh from the oven!

**Cooking time:** 35 minutes

# CHAPTER 5: Snack Recipes

## *1. Roasted chickpeas*

### Ingredients:

1 can chickpeas (drained and rinsed) - 2 tablespoons olive oil - 1 teaspoon cumin - 1 teaspoon paprika

- Season with salt to taste.

### Preparation:

1. Preheat the oven to 400°F (200°C).

2. Using a paper towel, pat dry the chickpeas.

3. In a mixing bowl, combine chickpeas, olive oil, cumin, paprika, and salt.

4. Spread them out on a baking sheet in a single layer.

5. Roast for 25–30 minutes, or until brown and crispy.

6. Leave to cool before serving.

7. Savour your crispy roasted chickpeas!

**Cooking time**: 30 minutes

## 2. *Vegan Trail Mix.*

### **Ingredients:**

1 cup almonds and 1 cup walnuts.

1/2 cup dried cranberries, 1/2 cup dark chocolate chips.

- Half-cup pumpkin seeds

### **Preparation:**

1. In a mixing bowl, combine the almonds, walnuts, dried cranberries, dark chocolate chips, and pumpkin seeds.

2. Toss until equally distributed.

3. Separate into snack-sized packs.

4. Seal and store for an easy grab-and-go snack.

5. Enjoy your nutritious vegan trail mix!

**Cooking Time:** Ten Minutes

## 3. *Guacamole with veggie sticks.*

### **Ingredients:**

-3 ripe avocados

- 1 juiced lime - 1 diced tomato - 1/4 finely chopped red onion - 1/4 cup chopped fresh cilantro

- Season to taste with salt and pepper. - Add carrot and cucumber sticks.

## Preparation:

1. In a mixing bowl, mash avocados and add lime juice.

2. Add diced tomato, red onion, and cilantro.

3. Season with salt and pepper, and mix to blend.

4. Garnish with carrot and cucumber sticks.

5. Eat your guacamole with vegetable sticks!

6. Store any leftovers in the refrigerator.

7. Ready in minutes for a nutritious snack.

**Cooking Time:** 15 min


## 4. Hummus & Whole Grain Crackers

### Ingredients:

- One can of drained chickpeas - Two teaspoons of tahini - Two tablespoons of olive oil - Two minced garlic cloves

- Juice one lemon - Season with salt and paprika - Serve with whole grain crackers.

### Preparation:

1. In a food processor, combine the chickpeas, tahini, olive oil, garlic, and lemon juice until smooth.

2. Season with salt and add paprika.

3. Serve alongside whole grain crackers.

4. Dip, crunch, and taste your hummus and crackers!

5. Store any hummus leftovers in the refrigerator.

**Cooking time:** 10 minutes.

## 5. Baked Sweet Potato Fries.

### Ingredients:

- two big sweet potatoes, peeled and cut into fries.

2 tablespoons olive oil, 1 teaspoon paprika.

- One teaspoon garlic powder.

- Season with salt and pepper to taste.

### Preparation:

1. Heat your oven to 425°F (220°C).

2. Toss sweet potato fries in a bowl with olive oil, paprika, garlic powder, salt, and pepper.

3.Arrange them equally in a single layer on a baking sheet.

4. Bake for 25-30 minutes, turning halfway, or until crispy.

5. Cool gently before serving.

6. Enjoy your roasted sweet potato fries with your favourite sauce!

**<u>Cooking time</u>**: 30 minutes

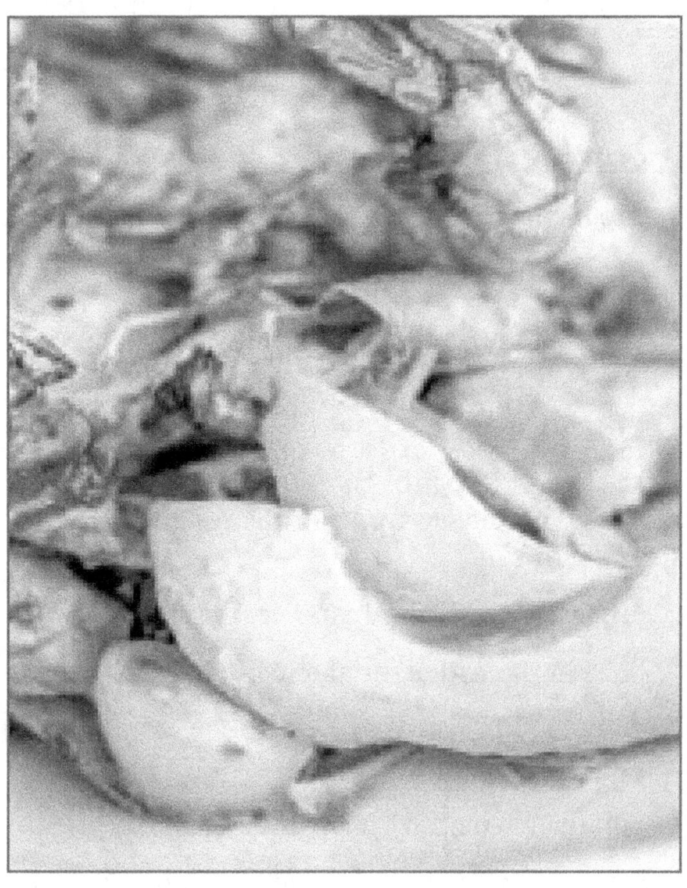

# CHAPTER 6: Desert Recipes

*1. Chocolate Avocado Mousse is vegan.*

**Ingredients:**

- 2 ripe avocados.

- 1/4 cup chocolate powder.

1/4 cup maple syrup, 1 teaspoon vanilla extract, a pinch of salt, and fresh berries for garnish.

**Preparation:**

1. In a blender, mix the ripe avocados, cocoa powder, maple syrup, vanilla essence, and a sprinkle of salt.

2. Process until smooth and creamy.

3. Place in the fridge for at least two hours before serving.

4. Transfer to serving dishes.

5. Finally, garnish with fresh berries.

6. Savour the thick and velvety vegan chocolate avocado mousse!

7. Serve cool.

**Preparation time:** 10 minutes.

## *2. Berry Muesli Crunch Bars*

### <u>Ingredients:</u>

2 cups rolled oats and 1 cup flour.

- 1/2 cup coconut oil, melted

- 1/2 cup maple syrup.

- 1 cup mixed berries (strawberries and blueberries) - 1 tablespoon chia seeds.

- 1 tablespoon of lemon juice.

### <u>Preparation:</u>

1. Heat your oven to 350°F (180°C).

2. To make the foundation, combine the rolled oats, flour, melted coconut oil, and maple syrup in a mixing bowl.

3. To make the crust, press half of the mixture into a baking dish.

4. To make the filling, blend mixed berries, chia seeds, and lemon juice in a separate dish.

5. Apply the berry mixture to the crust.

6. Crumble the remaining oat mixture on top.

7. Bake 25-30 minutes, or until the top is brown.

8. Cool before cutting into bars.

9. Savour your delicious berry muesli crumble bars!

**Cooking time:** 30 minutes


## *3. Banana Walnut Muffins.*

### Ingredients:

- Mash 2 ripe bananas - Melt 1/3 cup coconut oil.

- 1/2 cup maple syrup.

Ingredients: 1 teaspoon vanilla essence and 1 3/4 cups flour.

- One teaspoon baking soda

- One-half teaspoon cinnamon

- Half a cup chopped walnuts


### Preparation:

1. Heat your oven to 350°F (180°C).

2. In a mixing dish, combine the mashed bananas, melted coconut oil, maple syrup, and vanilla extract.

3. In a separate basin, combine flour, baking soda, and cinnamon.

4. Whisk together the wet and dry ingredients until just mixed.

5. Fold in the walnuts.

6. Spoon the batter into muffin cups.

7. Bake for 20-25 minutes, until a toothpick comes out clean.

8. Allow to cool before eating your delicious banana walnut muffins!

**Cooking time:** 25 minutes


# 4. Coco-Chia Pudding

**Ingredients:**

-1/4 cup chia seeds

- One cup of coconut milk

Topping: 1 tablespoon maple syrup, 1/2 teaspoon vanilla essence, and fresh mango segments.

**Preparation:**

1. In a mixing dish, combine chia seeds, coconut milk, maple syrup, and vanilla extract.

2. Stir thoroughly, cover, and refrigerate for at least 4 hours or overnight.

3. Re-stir before serving.

4. Transfer to serving glasses.

5. Top with fresh mango slices.

6. Savour your delicious, tropical coconut chia pudding!

7. Serve cool.

**Preparation Time:** 5 min

**Chill Time**: Overnight or 4 hours


## *5. Chocolate Chip Cookies are vegan.*

### Ingredients:

Combine 1 cup flour, 1/2 cup melted coconut oil, 1/2 cup maple syrup, 1 teaspoon vanilla extract, and 1/2 teaspoon baking soda.

1/4 teaspoon salt, 1/2 cup vegan chocolate chips.

### Preparation:

1. Heat your oven to 350°F (180°C).

2. In a mixing dish, combine melted coconut oil, maple syrup, and vanilla essence.

3. In a separate basin, combine flour, baking soda, and salt.

4. Mix together wet and dry ingredients, then stir in vegan chocolate chips.

5. Transfer spoonfuls of dough to a baking sheet.

6. Bake for 10-12 minutes, until the edges are brown.

7. Allow to cool before devouring your delectable vegan chocolate chip cookies!

**Cooking time:** 12 minutes

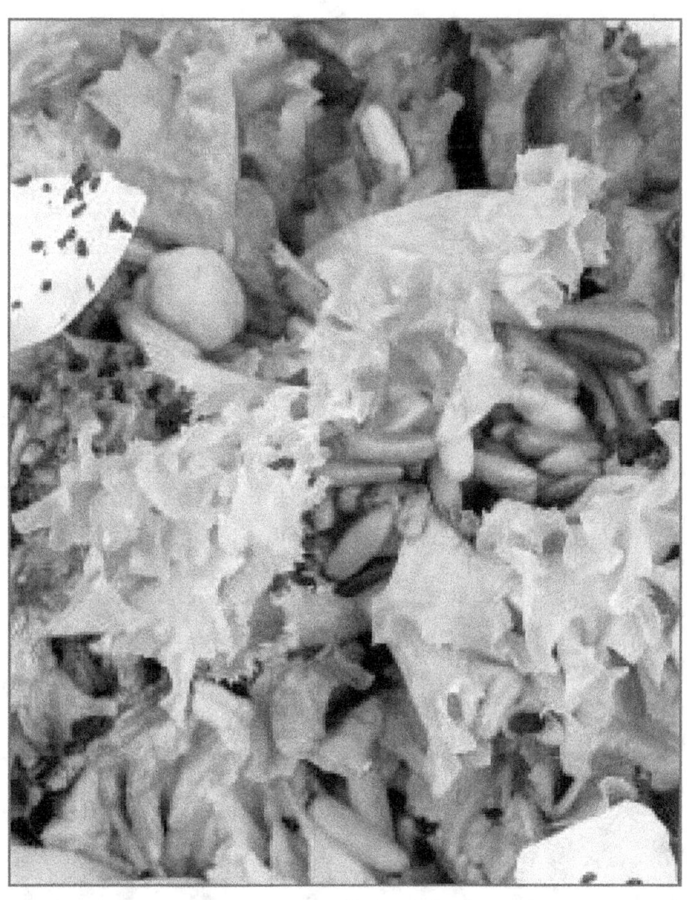

# CONCLUSION

In conclusion, this book is an excellent resource for seniors seeking to adopt a vegan lifestyle. It includes everything from nutritional suggestions to simple and tasty recipes for all meals. The step-by-step instructions make adjusting to a plant-based diet simple and pleasurable. More than just recipes, the book clearly explains the health benefits of adopting plant-based solutions. It's an uplifting and practical resource for seniors looking to live a healthier and more vibrant life, complete with useful ideas and colourful pictures. Whether you're new to veganism or searching for new ideas, this book is an excellent source of knowledge and support for seniors trying to live a full and joyful plant-based diet.

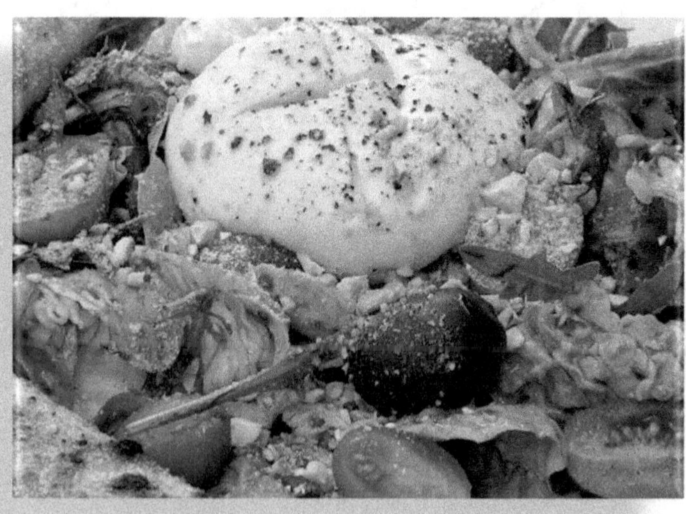

www.ingramcontent.com/pod-product-compliance
Lightning Source LLC
Chambersburg PA
CBHW050754250726
48662CB00005B/2225